FRENCH GRAPE SEED EXTRACT

Nature's Warrior Against Heart Disease, Inflammation and More

GAETANO MORELLO, N.D.

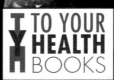

The purpose of this book is to educate. It is not intended to serve as a replacement for professional medical advice. Any use of the information in this book is at the reader's discretion. This book is sold with the understanding that neither the publisher nor the author has any liability or responsibility for any injury caused or alleged to be caused directly or indirectly by the information contained in this book. While every effort has been made to ensure its accuracy, the book's contents should not be construed as medical advice. To obtain medical advice on your individual health needs, please consult a qualified healthcare practitioner.

Copyright © 2017 To Your Health Books, Brevard, NC

Library of Congress Cataloging-in Publication Data is on file with the Library of Congress.

ISBN: 978-0-9961589-7-8

Cover and interior design: Gary A. Rosenberg
   www.thebookcouple.com
Editor: Kathleen Barnes • www.takechargebooks.com

Printed in the United States of America

10   9   8   7   6   5   4   3   2   1

Contents

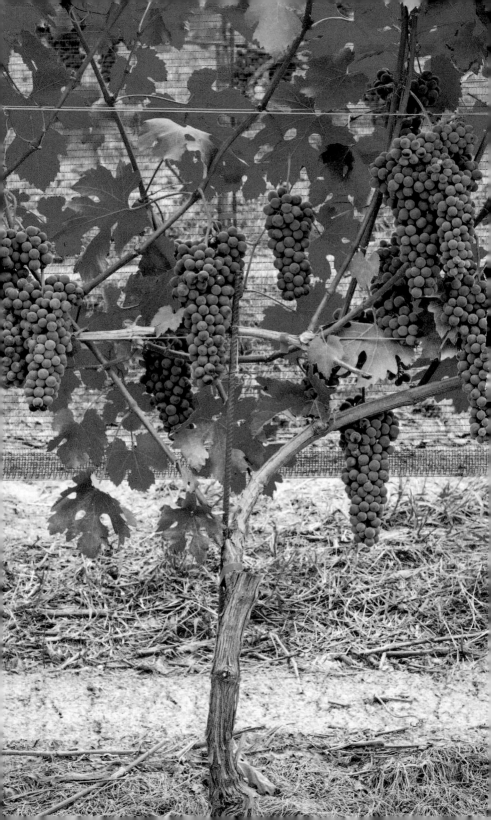

CHAPTER 1

Fruit of the Vine

Do you ever feel like you're fighting an epic battle against a host of health conditions?

Modern society tells us that as we age, we are likely to get heart disease, diabetes, cancer and, if we're lucky to live long enough, we could end our lives with dementia, sick and unaware of our surroundings.

Sometimes it feels like the lifelong fight against illness and disease is a losing battle.

While our culture may dictate that sort of thinking, be assured that the diseases of aging are not inevitable. DNA is not a destiny. What we do, the water we drink, the things we put in our bodies, the nurturing we receive and the environment we live in all dictate what we become.

By controlling our environment and lifestyle, we can prevent the "diseases of aging" from manifesting. The best method of being in charge of our environment is taking charge of what we put into our bodies

Yes, there is definitely a struggle to survive. However, there is a way of winning and it's simpler than you may think.

Dr. Christiane Northrup, once paraphrased a health goal first put forth by Abraham Hicks, author of *The Secret:* "Wouldn't you rather have your life end something like this: Happy, healthy, dead? Isn't that a lot better than being sick, decrepit and frail for years?"

Isn't that what all of us really want? We want a quality of life that enables us to live!

In fact, we are fortunate to have been given a wide variety of tools to retain vibrant health well into old age. These are the tools that can help create an internal environment fostering health and longevity.

Grape seed extract is one of those tools, a gift from nature. This is one of the most powerful disease-fighting compounds known to science. Grape seed extract is a warrior of unsurpassed power against disease and for life.

Extensive research has proven that grape seed extract:

- prevents and reverses heart disease

- kills cancer cells and prevents their return

- reduces inflammation

- improves blood sugar metabolism and blood sugar control in people with diabetes

- protects brain cells from the plaque associated with Alzheimer's disease

- speeds wound healing

- wipes out 10 disease-causing bacteria, including the deadly MRSA

- paves the way for longer life. (Yes, you read that correctly. Stay with me.)

We love wine and all that it contains

Millennia ago, our ancestors loved wine fermented from grapes and it seems that this tradition has withstood the test of time. Perhaps it is part of our genetic structure. Maybe there was—and still is—an intuitive sense of what is really good and life-giving for us. The seeds

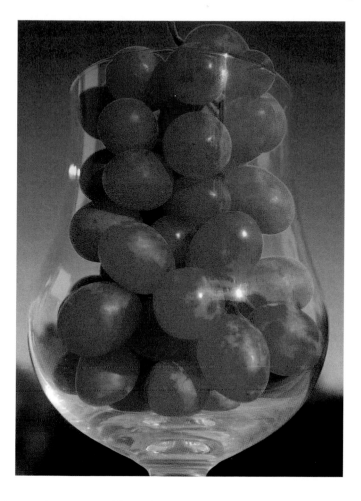

and skins of grapes yield not only a flavorful beverage, they contain unique substances that pack a powerhouse punch against disease.

The key lies in substances called oligomeric proanthocyanidins (OPCs). Although OPCs are found in many plants, they are concentrated to an extraordinary level in grape seeds, which explains their healing power.

OPCs are probably the most potent antioxidants known to science. What are antioxidants? An apple will turn brown after you cut it due to its exposure to oxygen; we can call this rusting. If you squeeze freshly squeezed lemon juice on it, it won't brown; the lemon juice acts as an antioxidant. Your lifestyle choices over the course of a lifetime and your exposure to environmental toxins cause "rust" (actually, the correct terminology is free radical oxygen molecules) to accumulate on your cells. That free radical oxygen exposure triggers chronic inflammation, opening the door to cell aging and genetic deterioration, paving the way for the diseases of aging, including heart disease, cancer, diabetes and more. All, at least 90 to 95% of our modern day diseases are caused by oxidative stress and inflammation.

Too bad we just couldn't squeeze lemon juice into every cell of our bodies, but there is something else we can do

The Great Neutralizer

Lab studies show that OPCs are much more effective than vitamin C and vitamin E and virtually any type of food in neutralizing free radical oxygen molecules. They are super duper lemon juice!

The antioxidant levels in grape seed extract are so high, they are quite literally off the scale. The ORAC (oxygen radical absorbance capacity) value of grape seed extract is so high, it is difficult even for modern equipment to accurately measure it. ORAC values are a measure of the free-radical fighting capabilities of a particular food.

We know that French OPC grape seed extract has an ORAC value of at least 2 million per 100 grams (3 ounces), higher than any other food! Compare this to blueberry, which has a rating of 6,552, dark chocolate powder at 40,200 and strawberries at 3,577. One attempt to measure the ORAC value of high quality grape seed extract failed when a meter went off the charts at an astounding over 15,000,000 per 100 grams.

Foods with high antioxidant power, like grape seed extract, balance immune system responses to reduce long-term (chronic) inflammation as well as short-term (acute) inflammation that govern wound healing and allergic responses.

ORAC VALUES (PER 1 GRAM)	
French grape seed extract	20,000
Ginger root	148
Elderberries	147
Cinnamon	131
Acai berries	102
Artichoke	94
Blueberries	47
Blueberries (raw)	96
Cranberries	90
Basil (dried)	61
Blackberries	59
Red wine (cabernet)	45
Sage (fresh)	32

—Source: U.S. Department of Agriculture, 2010

Of course, we are talking about the *right* grape seed extract. In recent years, there have been some really cheap products on the market that have little or no value. So-called grape seed extract from China can cost as little as $20 per kilo. In this case, you get what you pay for.

The best quality grape seed extract comes from tannin-free French OPC grapes that have a small molecular structure for the best absorbability—and the raw materials cost ten times as much. It's truly worth it, as you'll see as you progress through this book.

Disease Fighting OPCs and long-life resveratrol

There's an extra bang for your buck in grape seed extract.

Resveratrol is another antioxidant, this one using the power of polyphenols, also found in berries and peanuts. It's known for its unique anti-aging, anti-inflammatory and disease-fighting properties.

Studies show that resveratrol increases the lifespans of some animals (including yeast, worms, fruit flies, fish and mice) who are fed a high-calorie diet, but resveratrol seems to trick their bodies into "thinking" that they are consuming a life-extending low calorie diet.

We're sure that this longevity effect works in animals and now new research strongly suggests that this benefit extends to humans as well. That's great news for foodies and all of us who want to enjoy life and to enjoy a longer life!

All grape seed extract naturally contains resveratrol in addition to the powerhouse antioxidant OPCs. It's a two for one. That's a huge bonus!

Substantial research shows that resveratrol has many of the same disease-fighting capabilities as OPCs. It just works in a slightly different way. There is also evidence that the two combined, as they are exclusively in grape seed extract, complement each other synergistically, enhancing their total power.

A brief history

Despite the fact that humans have enjoyed grapes as food and drink for thousands of years, grape seed extract has only been heavily researched for about 65 years. And that research came about only in a roundabout way.

The tale begins with Jacques Masquelier, a French researcher who began working in the wine-producing Bordeaux region of France in the 1940s and 1950s. It might seem that the most direct route would have taken Masquelier straight to grape seeds, but instead, he took the circuitous route by looking at uses for the red skin waste from peanuts after they were pressed for oil. He began to look for other natural materials that contained OPCs and discovered pine bark extract was a rich source of those healing molecules.

His peanut research led Masquelier to a level of understanding of proanthocyanidins unparalleled in his time. He discovered that OPCs from red peanut skins shortened bleeding time, strengthened blood vessels and offered overall cardiovascular protection.

As a student of history, Masquelier was fascinated with the story of the sailors aboard the ship of French explorer Jacques Cartier. The winter of 1535 was particularly brutal, leaving Cartier and his crew stranded in ice on the St. Lawrence River. Left with little to eat except hard biscuits and dried meat, many of Cartier's crew died of scurvy before friendly natives showed them how to make tea from the nutrient-rich, reddish-colored bark of the pine tree *Tsuga Canadensis.*

Masquelier knew that this particular pine bark was rich in OPCs and it didn't take him long to discover another powerful source of OPCs right in his back yard—grape seeds. From this discovery, he pioneered the process of extracting OPCs from the grape seeds that were abundant in his Bordeaux region.

Today, grape seed extract has been deeply researched for its health benefits. As of this writing, the National Library of Medicine's database lists 934 published studies on grape seed dating back to 1997, including 39 clinical trials. (Since grape seed extract is a food and cannot be patented, few companies are likely to engage in this expensive investigation, so this number of human trials is uncommon and substantiates its value.)

Grape seed extract is a warrior of formidable strength in fighting the diseases of aging. For those of us who plan to live long, healthy lives, it should be a central part of our nutrient regimen.

My message to those of you who are already suffering from the degenerative inflammatory diseases of aging: Grape seed extract is essential to regaining health.

WHAT YOU NEED TO KNOW

- Grape seed extract is one of the most potent disease-fighting nutrients known to science.

- Science has proven that grape seed extract:
  - prevents and reverses heart disease
  - kills cancer cells and prevents their return
  - reduces inflammation
  - improves blood sugar metabolism and blood sugar control in people with diabetes
  - protects brain cells from the plaque associated with Alzheimer's disease
  - speeds wound healing
  - wipes out 10 disease-causing bacteria, including the deadly MRSA
  - paves the way for longer life.

- The healing power of grape seed extract is largely the result of its antioxidant and anti-inflammatory effects.

- The unique combined firepower of oligomeric proanthocyanidins (OPCs) in grape seed extract combined with resveratrol for an unbeatable one-two-punch against disease.

CHAPTER 2

Extinguish the Fires of Inflammation and Oxidation

Inflammation and oxidation are underlying causes of virtually every disease of aging. Stop those fires of inflammation and oxidation and you have slowed down the diseases of aging. It may seem a bit hard to swallow, but it's really as simple as that.

The inflammatory cascade

Let's start with inflammation.

There are two basic types of inflammation: acute inflammation and chronic inflammation. If you've ever sprained an ankle, whacked your thumb with a hammer or gotten stung by a bee (ouch!), the swelling, the redness and the heat are all part of the healing process. You are experiencing acute inflammation, an important component of the recovery process associated with an injury.

Background

When you get a tissue injury, your body's immune system sends out white blood cells to neutralize the inflammation. This is the human body's natural response to an injury. Your sprained ankle, bee sting or whacked thumb will hurt for a while, maybe requiring a little pain medicine or ice, and then it heals on its own, thanks to the warrior white blood cells and the innate healing power of the human body.

However, there's another type of inflammation that is far more insidious. Chronic inflammation is acute inflammation where there is no resolution of the injury. This is the type of inflammation that can be associated with pain as in the case of osteoarthritis. Often it has no outward signs of pain or no symptoms at all. It usually goes completely unnoticed as in the case of cardiovascular disease. Whether or not there is pain, they are both the result of inflammation.

When chronic inflammation continues unchecked, it disrupts biological functions, including the immune system. When this happens, the immune system can go into overdrive, constantly attempting to fight off those "foreign invaders," even though there is no real threat.

Chronic inflammation is almost always caused by lifestyle choices and by environmental factors including:

- eating processed and adulterated foods, especially sugar, excessive refined carbohydrates and vegetable oils

- overeating

- smoking

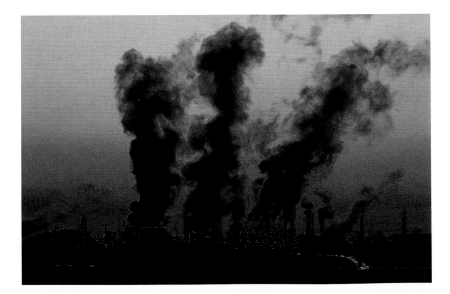

- breathing polluted air

- drinking municipal water

- using toxic personal care products (shampoo, soap, toothpaste, makeup, deodorant and more)

- toxic cleaning products

- petrochemicals and gas fumes

- pesticides and herbicides

- living and working in toxic environments (off-gassing carpets, furniture and bedding)

Let's add in one more cause of chronic inflammation: The Big S: STRESS. Long-term unrelieved stress, like most of us experience every single day, interferes with the ability of the stress hormone, cortisol, to stimulate the immune system and control inflammation, according to a 2012 study from Carnegie Mellon University. Researchers found that highly stressed people were substantially more likely to get colds when exposed to the cold virus as opposed to people whose lower stress levels promoted healthy immune function.

Beyond the higher risk of viral infections, unrelenting stress clearly opens the door to all of those diseases we want to avoid.

I'll say this in the simplest terms possible: If you are obese or have diabetes, heart disease, Alzheimer's disease or cancer, you have a disease triggered by chronic inflammation. These are lifestyle diseases. While you may not be able to control the air pollution in your town or the off-gassing furniture and carpet in your office, there are healthy lifestyle choices you can make that will minimize your risk of chronic inflammation, and the inflammatory diseases we all want to avoid.

If you don't have these diseases yet, paying attention to the lifestyle choices you can control and managing stress will go a long way toward protecting you.

And, of course, you can take grape seed extract. While nothing will 100% guarantee that you never get heart disease, cancer, diabetes or Alzheimer's, grape seed extract is one of the best life insurance policies the herbal world offers.

Oxidation

Oxygen is the key to life. If we are deprived of oxygen for even a few minutes, the consequences are grave, even fatal. So what is oxygen doing that makes it so critically important?

Oxygen is the substance that is solely utilized by the 1,500 or so mitochondria found in every cell of our bodies. These are the energy producing organelles that create the necessary electricity (energy) that allows us to function. The mitochondria are like hydro dams. The oxygen that flows through the mitochondria is like the water that falls down the dams and turns the turbines, creating energy. Imagine if we didn't have this energy production, we wouldn't be able to function

Another example: Everyone knows that cyanide is a deadly poison. Cyanide kills by interfering with oxygen's ability to flow through the mitochondria.

On the other hand, oxygen is actually a double-edged sword. Not only does it create the energy (electricity) needed for life, but it also produces oxidation.

We gave an example earlier, slicing an apple in half and watching the browning (rusting) caused from the cells on the apple's surface reacting with oxygen.

Think of rust on the bumper of your car—scientifically, it's caused by unstable oxygen molecules that are missing an electron or two. Unstable oxygen molecules, called free radicals, cause "rust" on your cells, damaging DNA much like they cause an apple to brown. It also causes cellular reproduction to be disrupted, so new cells are not exact copies of the parent cells. This is how aging cells open the way to vulnerable and diseased cell growth.

Our bodies are bombarded by free radicals 24/7. Toxins in air, food, water, cigarette smoke, industrial pollutants, pesticides, herbicides and other environmental toxins contribute to the free radical population explosion.

Yet, we are not helpless against this onslaught. Antioxidants found in plants, foods and nutrients neutralize free radicals and can even donate electrons to help stabilize these electrically challenged oxygen molecules and neutralize their destructive potential. Antioxidants like those found in grape seed extract are among the most powerful forces we have against free radical damage and disease.

Oxidative stress is the body's ability to combat those free radical oxygen molecules with antioxidant defense to keep the body healthy and balanced.

Andrew Weil, M.D., one of my favorite holistic physicians, says, "Health depends on a balance between oxidative stress and antioxidant defenses. Aging and age-related diseases reflect the inability of our antioxidant defenses to cope with oxidative stress over time. The good news is that with strong antioxidant defenses, long life without disease should be possible."

The Great Warrior quenches the fires of inflammation and oxidation

The best news is that we have control over both inflammation and oxidation.

Grape seed extract has hundreds of potent healing properties, but probably none are as important and as basic to human health than its ability to fight inflammation and oxidation.

Inflammation

It works as an anti-inflammatory in much the same way as NSAIDs (non-steroidal anti-inflammatory drugs like ibuprofen, naproxen and

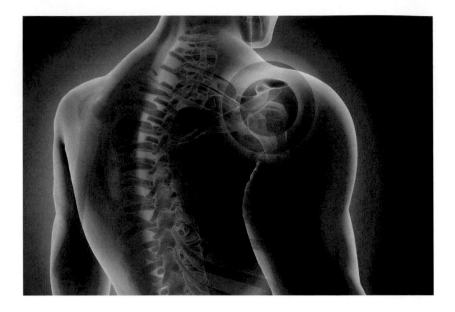

prescription drugs like Voltaren, Bextra, Celebrex and Vioxx) without the serious side effects that have been connected to these drugs.

NSAIDs are used to relieve pain related to inflammation, including arthritis pain. They also inhibit the COX-2 enzyme, which can lead to serious and sometimes fatal gastrointestinal problems as well as increasing the risk of heart attacks and strokes.

Grape seed extract has all of the anti-inflammatory benefits of NSAIDS and no negative side effects.

Research shows that OPCs prevent the body from manufacturing prostaglandins, the major inflammatory hormone that triggers inflammation as well as causing blood clot formation, the constriction of blood vessels and regulates the contraction and relaxation of the muscles in the digestive system and airways.

Oxidation

OPCs are highly effective free radical scavengers, interrupting the chain reaction of disease-causing cellular deterioration and repairs radical damage.

OPCs are formidable warriors against disease themselves with their stratospheric ORAC scores.

In addition to their own antioxidant power, OPCs can actually jump start the antioxidant, anti-clotting, anti-inflammatory and anti-tumor properties of the already formidable effects of vitamins C and E.

They also stop the formation of a Nuclear Factor kappa B (better known as NF-kB), one of the most powerful markers of inflammation that also controls cell survival and the programmed cell death that is necessary to keep the cells from dividing wildly and causing cancers and other disease and the duplication of DNA in cells (when that goes wonky, the cells reproduce imperfectly, causing a wide range of problems, including cancer).

I believe that the best grape seed OPC extract is one that can show a high ORAC value. ORAC values are a way of determining how much free radical fighting power a given fruit or vegetable has. While there's no way of duplicating the complex structure and synergy of a food, there are improved ways of taking some of the best components of fruits and vegetables and concentrating them to the point where you see extremely high ORAC values. The extract I recommend has an ORAC value of over 21,000 per gram!

WHAT YOU NEED TO KNOW

- Chronic inflammation and oxidation (free radical damage) are silent killers that are the underlying cause of virtually all of the diseases of aging: heart disease, diabetes, cancer and Alzheimer's disease.

- Since there are no identifiable symptoms of chronic inflammation and oxidative damage, there is no way to know you have that without medical testing—or until you develop one of the diseases they cause.

- Stress is a major cause of inflammation.

- Lifestyle choices, including what you eat, your exercise regimen and your exposure to environmental toxins can cause chronic inflammation and free radical damage to your cells.

- OPCs like those found in grape seed extract are among the most powerful warriors known to science to combat inflammation and oxidation.

CHAPTER 3

Pack a Punch
Against Heart Disease

Grape seed extract is no doubt your heart's best friend. Of all the considerable powers of this tiny seed, the prevention and control of heart disease is arguably one of its greatest strengths.

A study published in the medical journal *Lancet* in 1993 is foundational to today's knowledge of how OPCs protect the heart: Of 805 men studied by Dutch researchers, those who consumed the most flavonols (like those found in grape seed extract) had the lowest risk of a heart attack, and conversely, those who had the lowest flavonol intake had a very high risk of heart attack and an even greater risk of death from a heart attack.

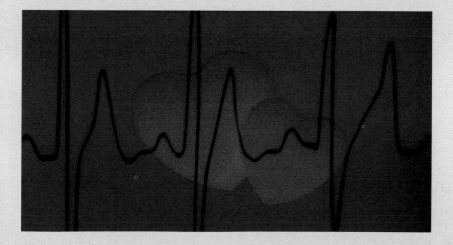

So, should we be afraid of heart disease? You bet we should, for all the grim statistics cited on the following page.

Is there anything you can do to prevent this onward march of death?

Absolutely!

Lifestyle choices are probably the greatest strategy for heart disease prevention.

Here are the simple ones that you probably already know, but you hope they don't apply to you:

Heart disease is the #1 killer for men and women in the world. The numbers are a bit daunting. They should be more than a little bit scary and they should get your attention:

- Cardiovascular disease (heart attacks, strokes and other cardiovascular disease) killed 17.3 million people worldwide in 2015 (the latest year for which statistics were available at this writing).

- By 2030, that number is expected to increase by more than one-third to 23.6 million.

- Although most of us think of heart disease as the product of a relatively opulent Western lifestyle, 80% of cardiovascular disease deaths take place in low- and middle-income countries.

- Cardiovascular disease is the cause of 30% of all deaths worldwide, one-third of all deaths in the U.S.

- It claims more lives than all types of cancers combined.

- Nearly half of all African-American adults have some form of cardiovascular disease.

—*Source: American Heart Association*

THE SUPER 7 STRATEGIES
TO PREVENT HEART DISEASE

1. Don't smoke!

2. Get moving! Exercise at least 30 minutes every day.

3. Eat less sugar, more fruits, veggies, whole grains and healthy fats.

4. Control your weight.

5. Control your blood pressure.

6. Control your cholesterol. Don't worry so much about lowering your cholesterol, be more concerned about lowering your triglycerides (blood fats) and increasing your HDL cholesterol. Note, that it's oxidized LDL cholesterol that is a contributing factor to heart disease (there is oxidation appearing yet again).

7. Control your blood sugar.

Now, I know that many of my readers have already heard all of the strategies above and you probably also know that #3—a healthy diet—has a heavy influence on four of the others: controlling weight, cholesterol, blood pressure and blood sugar.

I won't reiterate all of the sermons you've heard from your doctors or read in the press, but I can tell you there is a lot of truth here. It is worth your life to pay attention.

And adding high quality grape seed extract to your daily supplement regimen is a wise choice, too. Think of it as an insurance policy to the healthy choices you are already making.

Here's why: Numerous solid scientific studies show that grape seed extract covers four of the Super 7 strategies *plus* it helps prevent diabetes, a major risk for heart disease.

Grape seed extract lowers blood pressure

Probably the most exciting study of grape seed extract and blood pressure came from Italy, where 119 people with pre- or mild hypertension were given either 150 mg or 300 mg of grape seed extract a day. A control group was given diet and lifestyle recommendations with no assistance from any supplements or medications. The results showed both grape seed groups reduced their blood pressure substantially, but surprisingly, the lower dosage was more effective in reducing blood pressure than the higher dosage. In four months, blood pressure returned to normal in an impressive 93% of the lower dose group.

A similar study from the Illinois Institute for Technology confirmed the Italian study's results and found that grape seed extract lowered systolic blood pressure (the upper number) by 5–6% and diastolic (the lower number) by 4–7% with no negative side effects. As a bonus, they found the grape seed extract group had lower fasting insulin and improved insulin sensitivity, something important for people with diabetes who are also at high risk for heart disease.

An animal study from the University of Alabama at Birmingham attempted to mimic the increased risk for high blood pressure in women after menopause. In a University of Nevada study, grape seed extract protected rats fed a poor diet from high blood pressure and

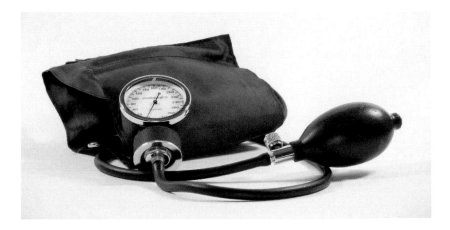

even seemed to neutralize the hypertensive effects of a high-salt diet. In addition, the grape seed extract seemed to enhance the animals' ability to neutralize those dangerous free radical oxygen molecules.

Grape seed extract strengthens and relaxes blood vessel walls

There is evidence that grape seed extract allows blood vessel walls to relax, allowing blood to flow freely through them with less force, further reducing blood pressure. It also helps activate an important enzyme called nitric oxide synthase, producing nitric oxide that relaxes blood vessel walls as well as regulating the production of the dangerous inflammatory protein NF-kB that can make blood vessels more rigid.

It also increases the production of collagen, the protein that connects muscles, bones, tendons and, yes, blood vessels. Why is this important? Think of a fire hose. If it's strong, it can withstand the intense pressure of the water that passes through it. Strong blood vessel walls are better able to withstand high blood flow and even high blood pressure without rupturing, as happens in certain types of strokes.

In simple terms, the OPCs in grape seed extract strengthen blood vessels while making them more flexible.

Grape seed extract reduces cholesterol and triglycerides

Grape seed extract turns out to be a formidable opponent of arterial plaque and elevated blood fats.

Excess cholesterol and elevated triglycerides can combine with fat, excess calcium and other substances in the blood to cause inflammation and eventually forming plaque. These fatty deposits in the blood vessels can eventually clog arteries, a disease called atherosclerosis, literally hardening of the arteries. Some blocked arteries may eventually rupture, causing a heart attack or stroke.

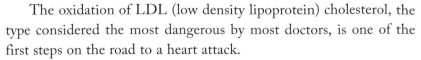

The oxidation of LDL (low density lipoprotein) cholesterol, the type considered the most dangerous by most doctors, is one of the first steps on the road to a heart attack.

Stay with me a moment—this gets a bit complicated:

A significant study from Georgetown University concluded that patients with high cholesterol (between 200 and 300 mg/dL) who took grape seed extract were able to reduce autoantibodies to oxidized LDL cholesterol by an impressive 50%. Oxidized LDL cholesterol is a particularly dangerous type of blood fat that has reacted with those free radical oxygen molecules we talked about in Chapter 2. When LDL cholesterol is oxidized, it produces long-term inflammation and tissue damage, and, in the case of heart disease, increases risks substantially.

So this Georgetown study is important to anyone with elevated cholesterol and even more important to people who already have been diagnosed with heart disease and/or diabetes (more about that in the next chapter) precisely because of its potent antioxidant properties to help neutralize this type of cholesterol.

A Spanish animal study confirmed the value of grape seed extract in treating high cholesterol. It normalized cholesterol in rats and even protected against fatty liver, an excess cholesterol condition related to obesity, among other things.

An impressive animal study from the University of Nevada at Reno showed how effective grape seed extract is at reversing the effects of high triglycerides (fats in the blood stream) that greatly increase the risk of heart disease. When researchers gave laboratory animals a super high fructose diet for 8 weeks, all their triglyceride numbers shot up a frightening 171%! But animals given the same diet plus grape seed extract actually *reduced* their triglycerides by 41%.

Before I get too far with this line of thinking, I do want to note that grape seed extract is not a magic bullet. Taking grape seed extract does not mean you can eat a terrible diet and neutralize all of the negative effects by taking this powerful supplement.

Grape seed extract reduces the risk of blood clots

In addition to the risks posed by narrowed arteries, blood clots contribute to the risk of cardiovascular disease. The two combined can be lethal.

Grape seed OPCs prevent blood clots, thus offering powerful protection against heart attacks and strokes.

Grape seed extract reduces blood levels of fibrinogen, the clotting factor, preventing clots from forming and dissolving clots that may already exist.

It is able to directly bust clots before they can form, according to a 2005 Japanese lab and animal study. A Polish study published in 2012 cited grape seed extract's ability to protect against clotting as part of its considerable antioxidant properties.

WHAT YOU NEED TO KNOW

- Heart disease is the #1 cause of death worldwide.

- Grape seed extract's impressive antioxidant and anti-inflammatory effects protect against heart disease by:
  - Lowering blood pressure
  - Strengthening blood vessel walls while making them more flexible
  - Lowering LDL cholesterol
  - Lowering triglycerides
  - Reducing the risk of blood clots that cause heart attacks and strokes

CHAPTER 4

Vanquish Metabolic Syndrome, Diabetes and Obesity

Metabolic syndrome, obesity and diabetes are an intertwined basket of health issues that add up to serious—and even life threatening–consequences.

Our modern lifestyle has mired us in these diseases. Much of our collective problem can be directly linked to the Standard American Diet (SAD) of high sugar and highly processed foods plus a sedentary lifestyle and unrelieved stress.

Read on to understand more and to learn how grape seed extract can help you overcome these dastardly health risks.

Metabolic syndrome

Let's start with metabolic syndrome, a collection of symptoms – or maybe better called health markers –– that can cause heart disease, stroke, and diabetes, if they are not addressed.

There are five conditions that the medical profession generally agrees comprise metabolic syndrome:

1. **Large waistline:** Belly fat is dangerous, pure, and simple. An apple-shaped figure and/or that dreaded beer belly are sure signs that you are at risk.

2. **High triglyceride levels:** If your blood work shows your triglycerides over 150 mg/dL, or if you are on triglyceride-lowering prescription drugs, you are at risk. What this means is that excess carbohydrate calories you consume are stored in your fat cells. There is some evidence that high triglyceride levels contribute to hardening of the arteries and, at extremely high levels, to acute pancreatitis.

3. **Low levels of HDL cholesterol:** HDL or the so-called "good" cholesterol is what you need to balance the effects of LDL cholesterol, which can increase the risk of heart disease. So in the case of cholesterol, the higher the HDL number, the better. In men, this is at least 40 mg/dL and women, 50 mg/dL.

4. **High blood pressure:** Elevated pressure of blood rushing through arteries can, over time, lead to plaque buildup as coronary artery disease, if your blood pressure is consistently over the ideal reading of 120/80 mm Hg. Medical science has recently adjusted those numbers to keep a "normal" reading of 140/90 mm Hg, although, I prefer that you keep your numbers in that lower range.

5. **High fasting blood sugar:** Even mildly high blood sugar can be a sign of early diabetes. Normal blood sugar when you awaken in the morning, before you eat or drink anything, should be between 70 and 100 mg/dL. Anything from 101–126 mg/dL signals impaired glucose tolerance and anything above 126 mm/dL is diagnostic of diabetes. If you know someone who has a blood sugar monitor, it's easy to do a nearly painless finger stick blood test. If not, your doctor's office can do it or you can have it done at any number of clinics.

If you have three or more of these risk factors, you have metabolic syndrome. The more of these risk factors you have, the greater your risk for heart disease, stroke or diabetes.

The *Journal of the American Medical Association* reported in 2015 that nearly 35% of the American adult population and 50% of Americans over the age of 60 have metabolic syndrome.

Obesity

Please read over the list of metabolic syndrome risk factors above. All of them are directly associated with obesity. As a nation, we are becoming fatter and fatter. And it turns out, it's not just a national problem. It's global.

More than one-third (34.9%) of American adults are obese, according to the Centers for Disease Control and Prevention (CDC). The epidemic is global. The World Health Organization (WHO) reported in 2008 that 35% of all adults worldwide were obese, and more worrisome is the WHO's statement that the number of obese adults around the world had doubled between 1980 and 2008.

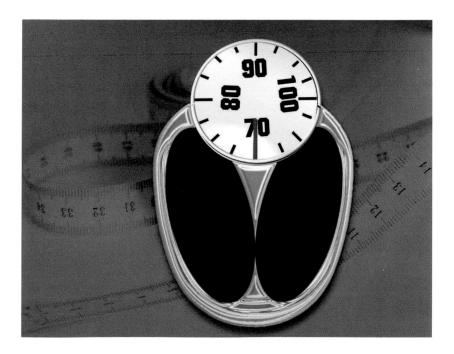

Add in the number of Americans who are overweight, but haven't quite tipped the scales to obesity, and you'll see that more than two-thirds of us have the excess poundage that puts us at risk of metabolic syndrome and a host of other diseases.

Not only does obesity increase the risk for metabolic syndrome, according to the National Heart, Lung, and Blood Institute, it also vastly increases the risk of heart disease, stroke, and diabetes. Sound familiar?

Obesity also increases the risk of cancer, especially colon and breast cancer, osteoarthritis, sleep apnea, infertility, and fatty liver disease.

The underlying causes of obesity and the ways to fight it could be the subjects of several books, but let me say that a healthy diet and active lifestyle could quite literally save your life.

Inflammation is part of the link here, which will become clearer when we start talking about grape seed extract in a few pages. Inflammation, the silent killer we learned about in chapter 2, is a huge cause of chronic diseases, including obesity.

Better lifestyle choices coupled with grape seed extract supplementation gives you a formidable weapon against obesity.

Diabetes

Type 2 diabetes was once called "adult onset diabetes" and was mostly the domain of people over 50. In recent years, that signature has been dropped because we've experienced an epidemic of obesity in children and teenagers, and the result has been a similar alarming rise in Type 2 diabetes among young people. More than 90% of people with this form of diabetes are overweight.

The increasing prevalence of Type 2 diabetes has closely paralleled the obesity epidemic with nearly 10% of the population (29.1 million people in 2012) with the disease, although 28% of them do not know they have it, according to the CDC. Worse yet, CDC researchers project that 40% of Americans currently alive will develop Type 2 diabetes in their lifetimes.

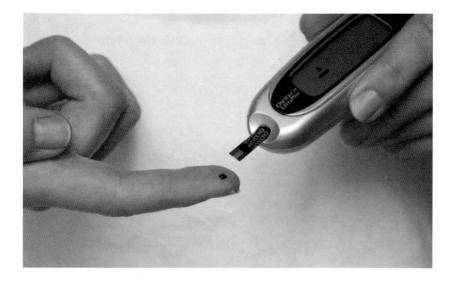

Type 2 diabetes, which occurs when your body can't use the insulin naturally produced by the pancreas (called insulin resistance), increases the risk of heart disease and stroke. Its other tragic side effects include blindness, poor circulation that can lead to amputations, kidney failure, impaired mental function, Alzheimer's disease, and more.

In people with diabetes, excessive blood sugar links to the flexible heart muscle like cement through a process known as glycation (AGEs – advanced glycation end products). This results in serious heart problems over time, including heart failure and heart attacks.

The Terrible Trio

Diabetes, obesity, and heart disease are so intimately connected that many doctors treat patients with any of these health issues as though they have all three. This often means they are given 6 or 8 or 10 or more prescription drugs, each of which has its own side effects requiring more medication to control. It's easy to see that this is a downward spiral that will eventually have fatal consequences.

All of this may seem overwhelming, but it doesn't have to be. Read on and learn how you can vanquish all three of the Terrible Trio.

Grape seed extract vanquishes the Terrible Trio

Yes, inflammation is a key underlying cause of obesity, heart disease, stroke and Type 2 diabetes, so it only makes sense that a powerhouse anti-inflammatory like grape seed extract would give the answers we need to vanquish the Terrible Trio.

But the Great Warrior goes much farther than that.

I believe that the single most important thing you can do is to follow a healthy eating plan and adopt a healthy lifestyle that includes a moderate amount of exercise, good sleep, and stress management in order to manage your weight and prevent diabetes. But it is abundantly clear that grape seed extract can help you get back to good health and stay there.

For example, a small, but important pilot study in Thailand found that people who ate a high carbohydrate meal and then took 300 mg of grape seed extract reduced blood sugar levels after a high-carbohydrate meal. The OPCs in grape seed can help stop the roller coaster of high and low blood sugars that lead to insulin resistance and, eventually, to Type 2 diabetes.

Two important animal studies from France and Spain, confirm that overweight hamsters reduced their waistlines dramatically with grape seed extract, even when they were fed a high fat diet. In addition, the grape seed extract reduced blood sugars, increased the ability to use insulin produced by the pancreas, and lowered blood fats—all important stepping stones to eliminate and prevent heart disease and Type 2 diabetes.

Further research confirms that grape seed extract can protect against damage caused by diabetes, including diabetic neuropathy that can lead to amputations.

In an impressive Saudi Arabian study, patients with fatty liver disease, commonly associated with obesity, were given 100 mg of standardized grape seed extract for three months. Their liver function and liver enzyme greatly improved, including severely limiting the number of fat cells that were able to infiltrate the liver, and positive effects were even seen in patients given only 50 mg daily.

And Chinese researchers found that grape seed extract has a powerful antioxidant effect against those dreaded AGEs (advanced glycation end products) that are at least partly responsible for the deadly link between diabetes and heart disease and other complications.

WHAT YOU NEED TO KNOW

- If you have three or more of the following: a fat belly, high blood pressure, high blood sugar, high triglycerides, low HDL cholesterol, you have metabolic syndrome.

- Metabolic syndrome puts you at a very high risk of developing Type 2 diabetes and heart disease.

- Obesity is a strong predictor of Type 2 diabetes.

- Type 2 diabetes is a strong predictor for all types of heart disease and stroke.

- Grape seed extract reduces belly fat, blood fats, blood pressure, and blood sugar, providing a simple and highly effective answer to these potentially serious health problems.

CHAPTER 5

Arrest Alzheimer's

Before we entirely leave the subject of diabetes, it's important to know that Alzheimer's disease has sometimes been called "diabetes of the brain."

Even in the earliest stages of the devastating memory destroying disease, the brain's ability to metabolize sugar is diminished. For decades, science has concluded that the characteristic amyloid plaques and tangles in the brains of Alzheimer's sufferers interrupt the delicate circuitry of thought transmission and memory.

The characteristic beta-amyloid clusters of proteins called "plaques" and clumps of dead and dying nerve and brain cells, called "tangles" are the generally agreed upon indicators that Alzheimer's disease exists.

Think of the brain's network of dendrites and neurons as an electrical system. Those plaques and tangles block the transmission of the electrical current or information through those circuits.

What's the link?

Many scientists now call Alzheimer's "type 3 diabetes." What's the link between Alzheimer's and diabetes?

Here are some things that science has proven in recent years that have advanced our understanding of this terrible disease:

 33

- We know that the risk of Alzheimer's is doubled in people with diabetes. Some studies say the risk is four-fold.

- We also know that insulin resistance defines Type 2 diabetes, sometimes called "diabesity," is primarily caused by eating too many simple carbs and sugars and not enough fat.

- We also know that insulin resistance starts the brain damage cascade.

- We also know that people with metabolic syndrome are at higher risk of pre-dementia and mild cognitive impairment.

- We also know that diabetes and Alzheimer's have parallel underlying causes: impaired insulin signaling, uncontrolled glucose mechanism, oxidative stress, abnormal protein processing, and the stimulation of inflammatory pathways.

- Finally, we know that the increasing and dramatic prevalence of Alzheimer's, diabetes, and obesity have been pretty much in lockstep since 1980.

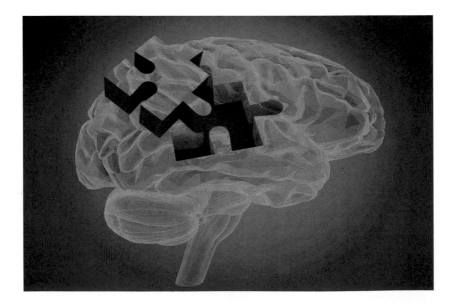

Does any of this sound familiar? Inflammation? Insulin resistance? Oxidative stress? We've talked about this in early chapters and we'll re-visit these subjects again and again in the coming chapters. At least one of these triggers is the underlying cause of virtually every disease we'll discuss in this book. Not surprisingly, grape seed extract powerfully addresses all of them.

Please re-read Chapter 4 on metabolic syndrome, obesity, and diabetes and apply all of the filters of what you've just learned about Alzheimer's disease to the science I've laid out here. You'll also see that grape seed extract addresses the underlying causes of the terrible Trio that now can be called the Fearful Foursome.

Grim statistics

The Alzheimer's statistics are grim. Alzheimer's and dementia cruelly rob the memories of 10 percent of 65 year olds, 25 percent of 75 year olds, and 50 percent of 85 year olds. It's now the seventh leading cause of death worldwide and researchers predict it will affect 106 million people by the year 2025. By the year 2050, the Alzheimer's Association reports, the number of people 65 and older with Alzheimer's will triple.

Patti Reagan, the daughter of President Ronald Reagan, coined the term "The Long Goodbye" in her 2011 book of the same title about her father's long battle against Alzheimer's.

It is a long and painful goodbye that takes a terrible toll on families. The average patient lives 10 years or more after diagnosis, growing more and more distant until the body still lives, but the mind is long gone. Only a shell of the loved one remains.

Yes, a small percentage of Alzheimer's is genetic, but I believe that most Alzheimer's is a lifestyle disease, just like diabetes. Control the symptoms of metabolic syndrome and you not only prevent diabetes and heart disease, in many cases, you can also prevent Alzheimer's.

Alzheimer's is considered incurable and irreversible. That may be true, but I'd rather dwell on the idea that Alzheimer's is preventable and that once someone has begun to slide down the slippery slope of memory loss, the deterioration can be slowed or even stopped.

Oxidation and inflammation

Since the late 1980s, research has handed out little hints that chronic inflammation hastens the Alzheimer's disease process and there are even some hints that inflammation may *cause* Alzheimer's.

There is no doubt that inflammation is an important factor in Alzheimer's, so it stands to reason that controlling inflammation will reduce the risk of developing the disease.

The same logic applies to oxidative stress from free radical damage.

Free radicals are the culprits in a number of biochemical processes that contribute to Alzheimer's, including the formation of advanced glycation end products (AGEs mentioned in Chapter 4), nitration or the constriction of blood vessels because of insufficient nitric oxide, and the accumulation of harmful fats in the bloodstream known as lipid peroxidation.

The above is a pretty fancy way of saying that free radicals certainly play a role in Alzheimer's.

Of course, antioxidants neutralize free radicals and even reverse the damage they cause. And you already know from Chapter 1, that grape seed extract is the most potent antioxidant known to science.

Addressing Alzheimer's and its underlying causes

Grape seed OPCs are at the cutting edge of Alzheimer's research. Research shows that grape seed OPCs:

- protect delicate brain circuitry to keep the "electrical" information flowing properly

- reduce the effects of oxidative stress (free radical damage) in the aging brain

- reduce inflammation in the brain

- protect nerve cells to prevent memory loss

- lower blood glucose to protect brain cells

A pivotal 2010 review of Alzheimer's research on grape seed extract from the Mount Sinai School of Medicine shows that grape seed extract stops the formation of those beta-amyloid plaques and tangles characteristic of Alzheimer's.

Probably the most exciting result of these studies is the confirmation that grape seed extract actually contributes to brain plasticity, the ability of the brain to adapt and create new neural pathways, effectively bypassing obstructions and damaged tissue.

Purdue University noted an interesting pattern: It seems that grape seed extract becomes more effective the longer you take it. The blood and brain levels of catechins and epicatechins, components of OPCs, were detectable as soon as someone took it, but they increased by as much as 282% over time with repeated doses.

Australian researchers found that lab animals given grape seed extract had as much as 44% less brain inflammation and 70% fewer plaques and tangles than animals that did not receive the grape seed OPCs.

WHAT YOU NEED TO KNOW

- Alzheimer's disease has sometimes been called "diabetes of the brain" or "type 3 diabetes" because of the devastating effect excess blood sugar can have on brain function.

- People with diabetes have at least twice the risk of developing Alzheimer's as people with normal blood sugar levels.

- Free radical oxidation and inflammation are important underlying causes of memory loss.

- Grape seed extract OPCs:
  - Protect brain cells, particularly brain cells circuitry
  - Reduce blood sugar
  - Reduce oxidative stress
  - Reduce inflammation
  - Enhance the formation of new neural pathways as alternative circuits for information

CHAPTER 6

Conquer Cancer

Cancer is the one word that probably strikes more fear in the human heart than any disease.

Sadly, more and more of us are hearing this devastating word every day as one in four Americans will die from cancer.

The National Cancer Institute projected that 1,685,210 new cases of cancer would be diagnosed in 2016 and 595,690 people would die of the disease.

There is a growing body of scientific evidence that cancer is largely a lifestyle disease. That's right—what you eat and how you live have a strong influence on the possibility that you will get cancer.

That also means that, to a great extent, you have control over your own risk of getting cancer. Yes, some cancers have genetic causes, but that number is very small: Heredity accounts for only about 5% of all cancers.

This isn't anything new. Since the days of Hippocrates, the concept of "We are what we eat" has been on the minds of holistically-minded practitioners.

The new field of epigenetics has validated this very premise. We do inherit genes, but the expression, what we call the phenotype, is triggered by the foods we consume, by the air we breathe, by the things we touch and in the nurturing we receive. In other words,

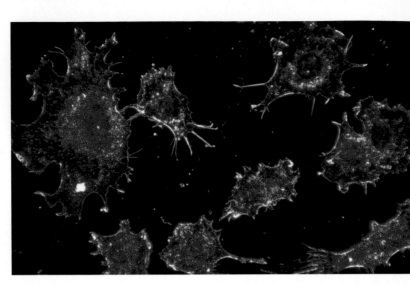

DNA is not a destiny: You get what your parents get because you do the same things your parents did.

This has been proven by the fact that even with all the medical advances and modern diagnostic tools, our cancer rates have not really been dropping. Since the War on Cancer was declared by President Richard Nixon 55 years ago, our overall cancer rate has decreased by only 5%.

Worse yet, the cancers that are most closely linked to lifestyle factors are *increasing* dramatically. Breast and prostate cancer diagnoses are off the charts—and the reasons may be more complex than it seems. However, diet is a major factor in both of these hormonally-related cancers.

The American Cancer Society estimates than half of all American men and one-third of all American women will develop some form of cancer in their lifetimes. Before you panic, let me add here that the *relative* risk of cancer depends greatly on lifestyle. For example, for all people who smoke, the risk of developing lung cancer is 2300% higher than for those who do not smoke. It's all back to the fact that it's not in your DNA, it's in the "triggers."

Case in point: As our consumption of fruits and vegetables and our daily exercise levels drop, our cancer risk increases. Add in the factors over which we have little control: air pollution, the presence of pesticides, herbicides and endocrine disruptors in virtually everything we eat as well as environmental pollutants like cleaning products and formaldehyde based furniture and carpeting used in homes, offices, and stores we visit and it becomes nearly impossible to avoid those environmental cancer triggers.

There is good news: Approximately 14.5 million cancer survivors are alive today. There could be more if we all followed a healthy lifestyle and included powerful antioxidant supplements like grape seed extracts in our daily regimens.

Grape seed extract attacks cancer from many directions

There is abundant scientific proof that a high quality diet rich in vegetables, fruits, healthy oils, whole grains, lean meat, and fish is the best cancer prevention strategy.

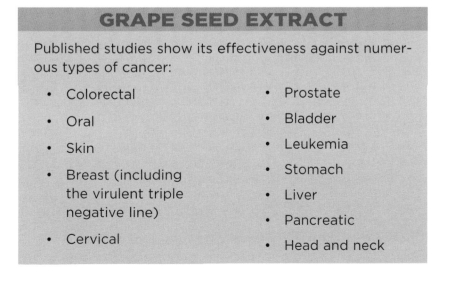

GRAPE SEED EXTRACT

Published studies show its effectiveness against numerous types of cancer:

- Colorectal
- Oral
- Skin
- Breast (including the virulent triple negative line)
- Cervical
- Prostate
- Bladder
- Leukemia
- Stomach
- Liver
- Pancreatic
- Head and neck

Clearly, we need to assemble all the forces we can muster to prevent and combat cancer as best we can. Grape seed extract shows a great deal of promise. It is one of the natural approaches to cancer with ingredients that doctors and patients should consider, and more importantly, to consume daily.

One of the reasons that grape seed extract may be so valuable in the fight against the development of cancer is that it concentrates beneficial plant compounds (the OPCs, polyphenols and flavonoids), which stop DNA damage. Research confirms that grape seed extract has a number of unique ways that could fight cancer that have put this compound at the forefront of cancer research.

Here's what the research on grape seed extract and cancer demonstrate:

May direct MicroRNA genes: At the risk of becoming too technical, let me say that grape seed extract targets MicroRNA genes. These tiny genes carry a tiny bit of extremely powerful information that lets them direct the behavior of thousands of genes around them. This is important because most cancers arise from genes that behave badly—either they go to sleep when they should be working to shut down mutations that lead to cancer or they work overtime to promote the growth of cancer cells. A study from the University of New Mexico shows that grape seed extract is very effective against lung cancer cells because of its ability to command those MicroRNA genes.

May stop cell changes that lead to cancer: In medical terms, this is known as carcinogenesis (the birth of cancer). Romanian researchers, looking at ways to combat several types of mouth cancer, found that grape seed extract neutralized the free radical oxygen molecules, which seems to be responsible for reducing the malignant cellular changes.

Impacts inflammation that has been associated with cancer: Grape seed extract stops the formation of inflammatory hormone-like substances called prostaglandins and was effective in killing lung cancer cells, according to research from the University of Alabama. Since thousands of studies have confirmed that inflammation is an underlying cause of virtually all types of cancer, this research holds great promise for grape seed extract for cancer patients, especially since it has no serious side effects.

Appears to tell cancer cells it's time for them to die: All cells have a finite lifespan, except cancer cells, which it seems are nearly immortal. The genetic signal that tell cells when their lives are over seems to go haywire in the case of cancer. The OPCs in grape seed extract awakens those signaling genes that tell cancer cells to die, especially when taken in large doses for people who have been diagnosed with cancer.

Italian researchers, whose published research journal indicated their skepticism, appeared to be impressed by grape seed extract's ability to encourage cancer cell death.

May inhibit tumor growth: Grape seed extract limits aromatase, an enzyme that converts androgens, the universal hormones, into estrogen in women. Since excess estrogen not balanced by other hormones contributes to breast cancer, the decreased aromatase levels prevent breast cancer and can also stop the spread of existing breast cancer, according to University of Alabama researchers. Breast and prostate cancer tissues typically have higher levels of aromatase. A study published in the journal *Cancer Research* discussed the valuable potential of grape seed extract, when their research showed that it slowed aromatase activity and reduced growth in MCF-7 breast cancer cells. They concluded, *"We believe that these results are exciting in that they show grape seed extract to be potentially useful in the prevention/treatment of hormone-dependent breast cancer through the inhibition of aromatase activity as well as its expression."*

Almost all women diagnosed with breast cancer are given a synthetic aromatase inhibitor called Tamoxifen. However, Tamoxifen

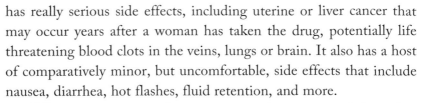
has really serious side effects, including uterine or liver cancer that may occur years after a woman has taken the drug, potentially life threatening blood clots in the veins, lungs or brain. It also has a host of comparatively minor, but uncomfortable, side effects that include nausea, diarrhea, hot flashes, fluid retention, and more.

Why not use grape seed extract, a natural aromatase inhibitor that has no serious side effects?

Protects smokers: Excessive wine consumption has been shown to contribute to the risk of several types of cancer, especially breast cancer.

The large California Men's Health Study of 84,170 men who were smokers came up with some surprising results: Men who were heavy smokers (more than a pack a day) reduced their risk of lung cancer by an impressive 60% if they drank one to two glasses of wine a day (up to 16 ounces). Whether this translates to grape seed extract (unquestionably a safer choice), will be determined by future research. In any case, it's not a reason to smoke, which has huge risks beyond lung cancer.

Smart targeting: The University of Colorado Anschutz Medical Campus has conducted some extremely important research on grape seed extract, including one study that shows this powerful healer has the ability to target specific colon cancer cells and stop them from growing and multiplying. Unlike chemotherapy drugs, grape seed extract can target cancerous cells without damaging healthy cells.

OPCs also help the liver to detoxify harmful forms of estrogen, reducing the growth of breast, stomach, colon, prostate, and lung cancer cells.

Stops angiogenesis: Cancer cells need a blood supply in order to have oxygen and nutrients that allow it to survive and grow. This process, called angiogenesis has been the subject of a great deal of promising research as a way to cure cancer: The theory is that if you can cut off the "food supply," you can kill the cancers and the growing tumor.

Grape seed extract is a powerful force in cutting off that blood supply that feed those tumors, according to several studies that show it interrupts the signals that form the blood vessels that feed tumors. Chinese research confirms it is the proanthocyanidins in grape seed extract that stop angiogenesis.

May target stem cells: Perhaps the most exciting research of all comes from Baylor University. We've all known someone who has had cancer and been treated, perhaps with chemo and radiation, gets better and is pronounced "in remission." Maybe even gets "well," only to have a re-emergence of a different kind years later. That is because cancer stem cells continue to live and circulate in the bloodstream, just waiting for an opportunity to take hold again and spread.

Baylor's lab research confirms that the OPCs in French grape seed extract kill colorectal cancer stem cells. It turns out that grape seed extract targets a unique pathway that supports the survival of these cancer stem cells. Researchers noted that this is "something that has never been shown before," and added they are "quite gratified and enthused" that this inexpensive treatment works in a way that no substance—pharmaceutical or natural—has yet accomplished.

Works with or without conventional treatment: Grape seed extract has a powerful effect on breast cancer cells when used alone or with a conventional treatment, according to another study from the University of Colorado. Their results showed that grape seed extract was extremely powerful against breast cancer cells, slowing their growth by up to 72% and causing 55% of the cancerous cells to die. Then they combined therapy with doxorubicin, a chemotherapy drug used to treat breast cancer and the effect was even more powerful. The two appeared to have a synergistic effect, enhancing each other's effectiveness, researchers concluded, opening the door to combining natural and conventional cancer treatments.

Helps those who choose conventional cancer treatment:
Grape seed extract has been shown to help the liver to detoxify from radiation induced poisons and chemotherapy.

Australian research also shows grape seed extract reduces the inflammation of mucus membranes in the mouth, digestive tract and small intestine caused by chemotherapy drugs.

In conclusion, it's easy to see how powerful grape seed extract is to target cancer from a number of directions. Most pharmaceutical drugs attack cancer from only one direction and carry with them a host of negative side effects, so grape seed and OPCs have formidable power against humankind's most-feared disease.

WHAT YOU NEED TO KNOW

- Grape seed extract and its OPCs appear to have the ability to attack cancer from many directions.

- It reduces the inflammation that is an underlying cause of cancer.

- Some studies show that it appears to stop some tumors from forming.

- When tumors have formed, stops the formation of blood vessels, affecting tumor growth.

- May stop cancer from returning by killing cancer stem cells in a way no other substances have been shown to work.

CHAPTER 7

On the Offensive
Against Other Diseases
and Conditions

This chapter will give us a new perspective on the powers of the Great Warrior, grape seed extract, to combat many other diseases and conditions.

It occurs to me that when we look at the big picture, the medicinal qualities of these humble seeds are indeed impressive.

In Chapter 2, we talked about inflammation and oxidation as underlying causes of almost all diseases of aging: heart disease, cancer, diabetes, Alzheimer's, and more.

Yes, some of the following diseases and conditions for which grape seed has been proven beneficial are related to inflammation and free radical oxidation—but not all. These are two key considerations in improving overall general health, however, there are some other unique ways that grape seed extract offers its healing powers.

We're learning more about grape seed extract's impressive powers against disease and promoting health nearly every day, so a compendium of its benefits will always fall short, but here are some of the best scientifically validated attributes of grape seed.

The body of research on grape seed extract and OPCs has expanded dramatically in recent years, with a total of 1,328 studies on these nutrients listed in the National Library of Medicine's database as of this writing.

Let's take a look at some of the other ways grape seed extract goes on the offensive against several serious diseases, illnesses, and conditions.

Antibacterial properties: It seems that grape seed extract is a natural antibiotic. Austrian researchers found that grape seed extract killed ten bacterial strains and other research confirms its effectiveness against antibiotic resistant *Staph* bacteria that can cause boils, cellulitis, food poisoning, and more. Another study confirms its effectiveness against 343 strains of *Staphylococcus aureus* (*MRSA*). What's more, Turkish research shows grape seed extract actually protects kidneys against the damage caused by the prescription antibiotic, amikacin.

Wound healing: Grape seed extract's ability to knock out bacterial infections certainly plays a role in speeding wound healing. Iranian research confirms grape seed extract's healing properties: People who underwent surgeries for the removal of moles or skin tags and given a grape seed extract cream not only had fewer infections, but were completely healed in 8 days, compared to people who didn't get the grape seed cream, who took 14 days to heal.

Venous insufficiency (leg swelling): This condition is caused by decreased strength and tone in the blood vessel walls that results in swelling, pain, itchiness, and tiredness, usually in the legs. A large Spanish review of studies on the subject confirms that grape seed extract reduces the swelling, pain, cramps, and restless legs associated with the condition.

Healthy eyesight/cataract reduction: The OPCs in grape seed extract are essential for healthy eyesight. They can reduce eyestrain and improve night vision by up to 98% by increasing blood flow to the eyes. OPCs in grape seed extract can also contribute to reducing the size of cataracts. Japanese researchers even found that grape seed extract prevented cataract formation in animals whose heredity made them particularly vulnerable to the condition.

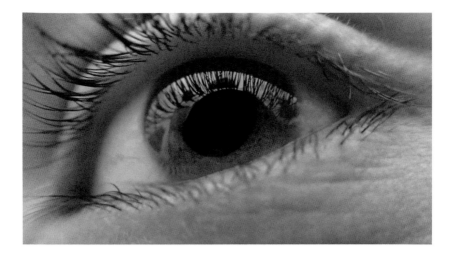

Allergies: Part of the power of OPCs is the anti-inflammatory activity. It turns out that grape seed extract is a natural antihistamine, reducing the sneezing and congestion commonly found in an allergic reaction. This natural antihistamine working with other anti-inflammatory powers, can actually stop allergic reactions, including hives, hay fever, and eczema.

Psoriasis and eczema: Grape seed extract appears to work in a similar way to ease the inflammation of psoriasis and slow the allergic reactions that cause eczema.

Attention Deficit/Hyperactivity Disorder (ADHD): A placebo-controlled, double-blind study published in the journal *European Child & Adolescent Psychology* found that after just one month, OPCs boosted attention span, caused a significant reduction of hyperactivity and improved motor coordination. The researchers noted that the symptoms returned one month after stopping the treatment, so OPCs would need to be part of an ongoing regimen. There is conjecture that grape seed extract increases the levels of blood vessel relaxing nitric oxide in the blood, helping increase mental focus. OPCs also regulate the enzymes that produce the brain chemicals dopamine and norepinephrine that help ease the nerve signals of hyperactivity. These findings have great potential for American children, who are being diagnosed with the disorder at alarming rates, ranging from a low of 5.6% of all children in Nevada to an overwhelming 18.7% of children in Kentucky in the past five years, according to the Centers for Disease Control and Prevention.

Arthritis: It goes without saying that the anti-inflammatory properties of grape seed extract and OPCs would significantly ease the pain and swelling of arthritis. But it goes a step farther in rheumatoid arthritis, an autoimmune disease that eventually destroys bones. Korean researchers found that grape seed extract slowed the destruction of bone cells and even stimulated the formation of new bone cells.

Fibromyalgia: The antioxidant and anti-inflammatory powers of grape seed extract help ease the pain and stiffness of this elusive disease and protect triggering muscle cells from damage.

Menopause symptoms: Hot flashes, brain fog, mood swings, insomnia, and more characterize the end of a woman's reproductive life. A Japanese study of middle-aged women in the early stages of menopause (perimenopause) showed that the women given either 100 or 200 mg of grape seed extract a day had fewer hot flashes, slept better, had less anxiety and depression, and lower blood pressure. An unexpected bonus: Their lean muscle mass increased in just 8 weeks, meaning they had less fat and better insulin absorption.

I think it is clear that grape seed extract targets disease from several directions, some of which we understand well, including inflammation and free radical damage, and others about which we are just learning. There is every reason to predict that the powers of this tiny seed will be even better understood in the coming years.

WHAT YOU NEED TO KNOW:

- Grape seed extract mounts a successful offensive against a wide variety of diseases and health conditions beyond its anti-inflammatory and antioxidant effects.

- It has been proven to kill a wide variety of disease-causing bacteria, including *Staphylococcus aureus* (*MRSA*) and speeds up wound healing.

- It relieves menopause symptoms and increases lean muscle mass in older women, helping them reduce fat and reducing the risk of diabetes.

- It helps children with ADHD to focus better and reduce symptoms of hyperactivity.

- It's a natural antihistamine.

- It relieves eyestrain and prevents cataracts.

- It helps re-build lost bones in people with rheumatoid arthritis.

CHAPTER 8

The Right Stuff

There is little doubt that grape seed extract is truly a "gift for health" from nature. It should be one of those important "special nutrients" you take daily.

Now here is the caveat in all this, not all grape seed extracts are created equal. I share this information repeatedly about botanical extracts with healthcare providers and the public at large to help them better understand the nutritional industry. Unlike pharmaceuticals, where the drug prescribed is exactly the same as the drug dispensed; in the nutritional industry this is often not the case.

There are numerous grape seed products available and they are not all created equally; they vary greatly in quality and price point.

Yes, you can buy "grape seed extract" for as little as 12 cents a serving. In this case, cheaper is absolutely not better. It can be money down the drain.

These inexpensive brands are made from a cheap Chinese grape seed extract that is minimally absorbable and therefore, have few of the health benefits attributed to this natural botanical in hundreds of published studies. By law, any extract that originates from grape seeds is considered a course of oligomeric proanthocyanidins (OPCs), but that is where the similarity ends.

Now, I'm not saying that the most expensive brands of supplements are always the best, but in this case, yes, it is well worth spending a little more—about 40 cents a serving—to ensure that your body can actually use the healing power of this incredible and well studied nutrient.

What's the difference?

First of all, absorbability is essential to any type of supplement. Whatever the nutrient in question, if your body can't use it, you're quite literally flushing your money down the toilet. Scientifically, it's called bioavailability.

Without question, you always want the most bioavailable product possible.

French grape seed extract comes from grapes grown in the wine regions of France, where some of the world's finest wines are produced. They are rich sources of polyphenols, abundant plant nutrients that are the underlying source of protection against all of the diseases we've examined in this book.

The ideal French grape seed extract is free of tannins. While those tannins give wine their body and flavor, they are not absorbable, so they don't provide any health benefits and you don't want them in your grape seed extract.

The OPCs in other forms of grape seed extract typically are composed of a variety of weights and sizes. The large non-absorbable molecules in grape seed extract are known as condensed tannins, which have no health benefits and are not absorbed by the human body.

Cheaper forms of grape seed extract are often spiked with additional tannins intended to bulk them up, resulting in low prices and virtually no health benefits.

Look for a tannin-free product with a small molecular structure for maximum absorption.

The best product has 99% polyphenols, 80% OPCs and 27–32% dimers.

If that sounds like a complicated search, let me reassure you that

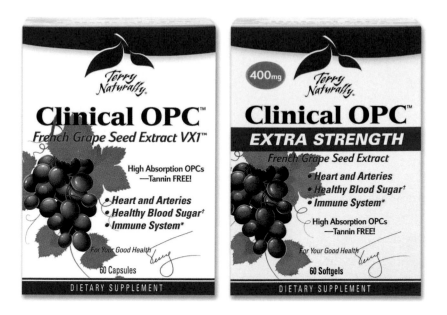

it's not complicated at all. Remember, what we discussed earlier: A key component is learning about the brands that offer the high quality, studied material that back the clinical research. A product that meets these requirements is Terry Naturally Clinical OPC™, a company that remains at the forefront of innovative nutritional ingredients of the highest quality.

It's important to learn about the companies that are doing things to improve people's well being. This is one of those companies offering "true" health solutions.

This product comes in 150 mg and 400 mg formulations plus a special super combination with curcumin that we'll need to discuss shortly.

In the meantime, here is a list of recommended dosages for conditions grape seed extract can address. Obviously, you should always be under the care of a physician and/or a holistically oriented physician with a background and an understanding of scientifically validated nutritional ingredients.

- Support proper blood pressure: 150–300 mg daily
- Cancer Support: 400–1200 mg daily
- Help in supporting cancer prevention: 150–400 mg daily
- Support chronic venous insufficiency (legs): 150–300 mg daily

One-two punch

Grape seed is unquestionably one of the most formidable foes of chronic disease.

Curcumin is one of the most studied natural ingredients in the world, with probably the greatest intrinsic effect of any natural ingredient I've used in clinical practice.

I've been combining ingredients with supportive effects for several years.

Like any practicing physician, I make my best effort combined with lots of homework searching for the most effective ingredients for my patients.

Although I've used a number of different types of curcumin-based extracts, BCM-95 continues to provide consistent outcomes with my patients. To date, I have prescribed this unique curcumin to over 1,000 patients with measurable outcomes on a variety of conditions. The anti-inflammatory effects are excellent and the clinical research supports this observation.

In 2012, a randomized, pilot study was carried out to assess the effectiveness and safety of BCM-95 in patients with active rheumatoid arthritis. The results showed better benefits in the patients taking BCM-95 than those taking the anti-inflammatory pharmaceutical, diclofenac. This is remarkable since the BCM-95 has no side effects.

Another study published in *Phytotherapy Research* in 2016 showed curcumin BCM-95's positive outcomes in reducing the symptoms of depression. There are numerous other studies done, in progress or planned all over the world on Alzheimer's disease, various types of

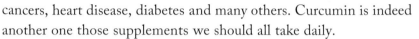

cancers, heart disease, diabetes and many others. Curcumin is indeed another one those supplements we should all take daily.

An obvious combination would be OPCs with BCM-95. Wouldn't this make a phenomenal daily supplement? Just looking at the ORAC antioxidant power of these two ingredients is remarkable with BCM-95 hitting 1.5 million per 100 grams while grape seed extract comes in at 2 million per 100 grams.

The good news: OPCs and BCM-95 are available in combination form!

If you take the time to just look at the robust research on these two ingredients, the positive impact their mechanisms of action can have on the human body, you will be convinced that these should become part of your daily supplement regimen.

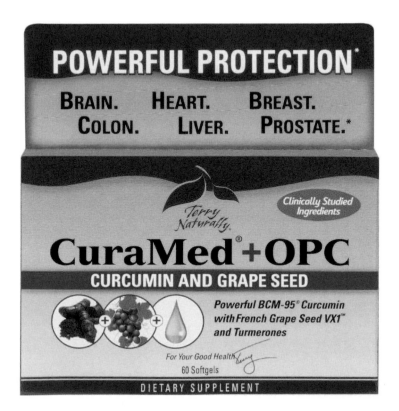

Finally...

As a practicing naturopathic doctor with a private practice, and the only naturopathic doctor working at a major hospital in North America, I am extremely careful when I select products that I prescribe for my patients. Poor quality products that may or may not be of benefit and could actually cause harm cannot jeopardize the health of my patients and my reputation. Our premise is "to do no harm," but at the same time recommend nutritional supplements that provide measurable outcomes.

My recommendations are without biases; I recommend the best possible ingredients for the desired outcome. So it is important to understand brands and what brands provide the best possible product for the discussed health concern.

In this book, I have introduced you to a powerful natural product, French grape seed extract, sold under the brand name Clinical OPC™. This form of grape seed extract has been proven to be much more effective than widely available cheap alternative grape seed extracts that are poorly absorbed by the human body, so they have little effectiveness.

French grape seed extract—the VX1 formulation—has been clinically proven to be highly effective because it only contains the very low weight molecules that are 100% absorbable.

If you supplement your nutritional program with a tannin-free French grape seed extract such as Clinical OPC™, you will notice the results in a few months or less.

In my experience, these natural ingredients can have impressive long-term benefits. They are free from the side effects and complications caused by pharmaceuticals. More and more physicians are beginning to see that the side effects of drugs often outweigh their benefits.

Natural products are made up of hundreds of molecules that work on multiple pathways in the body at multiple levels of those pathways, all simultaneously. It's like having a pharmacy in a bottle without the fear of side effects. Drugs are limited to what they can accomplish as they are only made up of one molecule targeting one pathway in the body, therefore, throwing many other pathways out of balance, and the benefits are limited as well.

My passion is to educate you, the reader and my patients, to the powerful effects of natural products that can alleviate sickness and suffering without doing harm.

Include these products: Clinical OPC™ and CuraMed®+OPC in your nutritional regimen. They are sure to pay off huge health benefits.

From literally thousands of studies on grape seed extract and curcumin, I have come to the conclusion that almost everyone should take them together every day.

Healthy regards,
Dr. Gaetano Morello, N.D.
Vancouver, British Columbia • September 2016

References

Chapter 1: Fruit of the Vine

ORAC table download: www.ars.usda.gov/nutrientdata/ORAC

Sinclair DA. Toward a unified theory of caloric restriction and longevity regulation. *Mechanics of Ageing and Development.* 2005 Sep;126(9):987–1002.

Baur JA, Pearson KJ, Price NL, et al. Resveratrol improves health and survival of mice on a high-calorie diet. *Nature.* 2006 Nov 16;444(7117):337–42.

Sovak M. Grape extract, resveratrol, and its analogs: a review. *Journal of Medicinal Food.* 2001;4(2):93–105.

Chapter 2: Extinguish the Fires of Inflammation and Oxidation

Cohen S, Janick-Deverts D et al. Chronic Stress, glucocortisoid receptor resistance, inflammation and disease risk. *Proceedings of the National Academy of Sciences USA.* 2012 Apr 17;109(16):5995–99. doi: 10.1073/pnas.1118355109.

Facino RM, et all. Free radicals scavenging action and anti-enzyme activities of Proanthocyanadins from Vitis vinifera. *Arzneim Forsch,* 1994; 44: 592–601.

Terra, X, Valls, J et al. Grape-Seed Procyanidins Act as Antiinflammatory Agents in Endotoxin-Stimulated RAW 264.7 Macrophages by Inhibiting NFkB Signaling Pathway. *Journal of Agricultural and Food Chemistry;* 4357–65.

Das, S, Das, D. Anti-Inflammatory Responses of Resveratrol. *Inflammation & Allergy-Drug Targets IADT* 2007; 168–173.

Chapter 3: Pack a Punch Against Heart Disease

Hertog MG, Feskens EJ et al. Dietary antioxidant flavonoids and risk of coronary heart disease: the Zutphen Elderly Study. *Lancet;* 1993 Oct 23;342(8878):1007–11.

Belcaro G et al. Grape seed procyanidins in pre- and mild hypertension: a registry study. *Evidence-Based Complementary and Alternative Med;* 2013;2013: 313142. ?

Carlson S, Peng N et al. The effects of botanical dietary supplements on cardiovascular, cognitive and metabolic function in males and females. *Gender Medicine;* 2008; 5(SuppA);S76–S90.

Park E, Edirisinsghe I et al. Effects of grape seed extract beverage on blood pressure and metabolic indices in individuals with pre-hypertension: a randomised, double-blinded, two-arm, parallel, placebo-controlled trial. *British Journal of Nutrition;* 2016 Jan 28;115(2):226–238. doi: 10.1017/S0007114515004328.

Fitzpatrick DF et al. Vasodilating procyanidins derived from grape seeds. Annals of the New York Academy of Sciences; 2002; 957:78–89. *LoS One;* 2015 Oct 12;10(10):e0140267.

Downing LE, Heidker RM et al. A Grape Seed Procyanidin Extract Ameliorates Fructose-Induced Hypertriglyceridemia in Rats via Enhanced Fecal Bile Acid and Cholesterol Excretion and Inhibition of Hepatic Lipogenesis. *LoS One;* 2015 Oct 12;10(10):e0140267.

Preuss HG, Wallerstedt D et al. Effects of niacin-bound chromium and grape seed proanthocyanidin extract on the lipid profile of hypercholesterolemic subjects: a pilot study. *Journal of Medicine;* 2000;31(5–6):227–246.

Sano T, Oda E et al. Anti-thrombotic effect of proanthocyanidin, a purified ingredient of grape seed. *Thrombosis Research;* 2005;115(1–2):115–121.

Chapter 4: Vanquish Diabetes and Obesity

Aguilar M, Bhuket T et al. Prevalence of the metabolic syndrome in the United States, 2003–2012. *Journal of the American Medical Association;* 2015;May 19;313(19):1973–74.

Sung, KC, Rhee EJ et al. Increased Cardiovascular Mortality in Subjects With Metabolic Syndrome Is Largely Attributable to Diabetes and Hypertension in 159,971 Korean Adults. *Journal of Clinical Endocrinology and Metabolism;* 2015 Jul;100(7):2606–12.

Ogden, CL, Carroll MD et al. Prevalence of Overweight and Obesity in the United States, 1999–2004. *Journal of the American Medical Association;* 2006;295(13):1549–55.

Sapwarobol S, et al. Postprandial blood glucose response to grape seed extract in healthy participants: A pilot study. *Pharmacogn Mag.* ?2012;8(31):192–196. *Pharmacognosy Magazine;* 2012 Jul;8(31):192–196.

Baskaran Yogalakshmi, Saravanan Bhuvaneswari, S Sreeja, Carani Venkatraman Anuradha. Grape seed proanthocyanidins and metformin act by different mechanisms to promote insulin signaling in rats fed high calorie diet. *Journal of Cell Communication and Signaling;* 2013 Sep 12.

Caimari A, del Bas JM et al. Low doses of grape seed procyanidins reduce adiposity and improve the plasma lipid profile in hamsters. *International Journal of Obesity* (London);2013 Apr;37(4):576–583.

Chapter 5: Arrest Alzheimer's

Campos-Pena V, Toral-Rios D et al. Metabolic syndrome as a risk factor for Alzheimer's disease: is A[beta] a crucial factor in both pathologies? *Antioxidants and Redox Signaling;* 2016 Jul 1. [Epub ahead of print]

Rani V, Deshmukh R et al. Alzheimer's disease: Is this a brain specific diabetic condition? *Physiology and Behavior;* 2016 May 25;164(Pt A):259–267.

Wang J, Bi W et al. Targeting multiple pathogenic mechanisms with polyphenols for the treatment of Alzheimer's disease-experimental approach and therapeutic implications. *Frontiers in Aging Neuroscience;* 2014 Mar 14;6:42.

Perry G, Cash A et al. Alzheimer Disease and Oxidative Stress. *Journal of Biomedicine and Biotechnology;* 2002;2(3):120–123.

Pasinetti G, Ho L. Role of grape seed polyphenols in Alzheimer's disease neuropathology. *Nutrition and Dietary Supplements;* 2010 Aug 1; 2010(2): 97–103.

Wang YJ, Thomas P et al. Consumption of grape seed extract prevents amyloid-beta deposition and attenuates inflammation in brain of an Alzheimer's disease mouse. *Neurotoxicology Research;* 2009 Jan;15(1):3–14.

Feruzzi MG, Lobo JK et al. Bioavailability of gallic acid and catechins from grape seed polyphenol extract is improved by repeated dosing in rats: implications for treatment in Alzheimer's disease. *Journal of Alzheimer's Disease;* 2009;18(1):113–124

Chapter 6: Conquer cancer

Toden S, Goel A. Novel and previously unknown mechanisms of action by which low molecular weight oligomeric proanthocyanins (OPCs) from French Grape Seed Extract VX1 help eradicate colorectal cancer cells. Oligomeric proanthocyanidins inhibit Hippo-YAP pathway and prevent colorectal cancer stem cell formation. Poster presentation at the annual American Association for Cancer Research (AACR) meeting. New Orleans, LA. April 16–20, 2016.

Mao JT, Xue B et al. MicroRNA-19a/b mediates grape seed procyanidin extract-induced anti-neoplastic effects against lung cancer. *Journal of Nutritional Biochemistry.* 2016 May 20;34:118–125.

Scrobata I, Bolfa P et al. Natural chemopreventive alternatives in oral cancer chemoprevention. *Journal of Physiology and Pharmacology;* 2016 Feb;67(1):161–172.

Derry M, Raina K et al. Differential effects of grape seed extract against human colorectal cancer cell lines: The intricate role of ?death receptors and mitochondria. *Cancer Letters.* 2012 Dec 23.

Sharma G, Tyagi AK et al. Synergistic anti-cancer effects of grape seed extract and conventional cytotoxic agent ?doxorubicin against human breast carcinoma cells. *Breast Cancer Research and Treatment;* 2004 May;85(1):1–12.

Sharma SD, Meeran Sm et al. Proanthocyanidins inhibit in vitro and in vivo growth of human non-small cell lung cancer cells by inhibiting the prostaglandin E(2) receptors. *Molecular Cancer Therapy;* 2010 Mar;9(3):569–580.

Dinicola S, Cucina A et al. Apoptosis-inducing factor and caspase-dependent apoptotic pathways triggered by different grape seed extracts on human colon cancer cell line Caco-2. *British Journal of Nutrition;* 2010 Sep;104(6):824–832.

Chao C, Slezak JM et al. Alcoholic beverage intake and risk of lung cancer: the California Men's Health Study. *Cancer Epidemiology, Biomarkers and Prevention;* 2008 Oct;17(10):2692–99.

Chapter 7: On the Offensive Against Other Diseases and Conditions

Mayer R et al. Proanthocyanidins: target compounds as antibacterial agents. *Journal of Agriculture and Food Chemistry;* 2008;56(16):6959–66.

Al-Habib A, et al. Bactericidal effect of grape seed extract on methicillin-resistant Staphylococcus aureus (MRSA). *Journal of Toxicological Sciences;* ?2010;35(3):357–64.

Hemmati AA, Foroozan M et al. The topical effect of grape seed extract 2% cream on surgery wound healing. *Global Journal of Health Science;* 2014 Oct 29;7(3):52–58.

Martinez-Zapata MJ, Vernooii RW et al. Phlebotonics for venous insufficiency. *Cochrane Database of Systematic Reviews;* 2016 Apr 6;4:CD003229.

About the Author

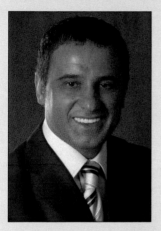

Dr. Gaetano Morello is a licensed naturopathic physician practicing in Vancouver, Canada.

Since 1991, Dr. Morello has been training and educating physicians, pharmacists and health experts on the scientific use of natural medicines. Contributing author to the authoritative text on alternative medicine, *A Textbook of Natural Medicine,* he is also author of *Whole Body Cleansing, Cleanse An Inside Out Approach.*

As a member of the Quality Assurance Committee for the College of Naturopathic Physicians of British Columbia, Dr. Morello's mission is to ensure that naturopathic medicine utilizes the highest level of quality care for all patients.

Dr. Morello is a clinician at the Complex Chronic Disease Program at BC Women's Hospital in Vancouver, treating chronic fatigue syndrome, fibromyalgia, myalgic encephalomyelitis and Lyme disease.

He is the first naturopathic physician to hold such a position at a major North American hospital.

Index